Table of Contents

The Efficacy of Antacids in Treating Gastroenteritis

1. Introduction to Gastroenteritis

Causes include most commonly viral or bacterial pathogens, such as with viral gastroenteritis. Transmission is commonly via diarrhea, vomiting, or fecally contaminated hands of person-to-person outbreaks, and the ingestion of fecally contaminated food or water. Risk factors for this condition include a weakened immune system, having been exposed to another individual with the illness (as is common in institutional settings and among travelers), poor hygiene, lack of access to clean water, and travel or camping in the wilderness. The disease is often self-limiting (improves without any treatment); however, if supportive care is not provided, electrolyte imbalances may result. Water loss and, if severe, metabolic acidosis can occur due to the vomiting and diarrhea. This is particularly important in children, the elderly, and those with other health problems when dehydration is debilitating.

Gastroenteritis is the inflammation of the lining of the stomach and intestines and occurs mainly due to a viral or bacterial infection. It is one of the most common disease conditions. Gastroenteritis is the inflammation of the stomach and intestines, typically causing nausea, vomiting, diarrhea, and fever. Other, less common, causative factors may include parasites, fungal infections, food allergies or toxicities, and relatively rarely, adverse reactions to medications or radiation therapy. The most common symptoms of diarrhea are abdominal bloating or cramps, thin stools, stool changes, fecal incontinence, mucus present in the stool, or watery stool.

1.1. Definition and Symptoms

A few of gastroenteritis's key symptoms include nausea, which is a fever-producing illness that triggers a feeling of discomfort at the sternocostal angle, which is the place at the base of the sternum where the ribs meet the breastbone. Vomiting, or expelling foods, fluids, and other intestinal substances or juices may occur. Diarrhea, which is a higher frequency, carrying loose, moist, or watery fecal matter (watery feces, known as "runny tummy", "Sultan's sickness", or "barking stomach" in the case of diarrhea). In most instances, the cumulative frequency of germs is halted or minimized in the abdomen, and the individual's signs and symptoms are treated with antacids to minimize the acidity of the ill individual's stomach and increase the pH of the abdomen in order to help treat gastroenteritis. The pH of the stomach can be determined by the hydronium ion, which is secreted by parietal cells in the lining of the stomach. Antacids neutralize the excess acidity in the stomach and encourage the stomach to produce smaller amounts of hydrochloric acid, which has little effect on protein digestion in the stomach. If an antacid bottle specifies gastrointestinal (GI) distress or an uncomfortable stomach, it is usually common to use antacids for gastroenteritis in these circumstances.

Gastroenteritis is a disorder characterized by irritation and inflammation of the stomach and the intestines. The suffix "-itis" is used, which comes from the Greek word "ito" or "a". It denotes inflammation, so that the name gastroenteritis denotes irritation of the stomach.

Gastroenteritis is a nonspecific manifestation; it is primarily identified as dyspepsia, meaning indigestion, when the abdomen feels full, and belching takes place.

1.2. Causes and Risk Factors

Moreover, the potential for an antacid medication to attenuate gastroenteritis symptoms is quite promising, not only scientifically in theory but also in terms of public health. If it can be shown that using an antacid proves to lessen the harsh symptoms frequently associated with gastroenteritis such as diarrhea or vomiting, it has the potential to positively impact those people who are susceptible to developing this disease for various reasons. Crucially, this research has direct application to the target population, with the choice of a rather innocuous drug – an antacid – minimizing any potential risks associated with its use by a community suffering from gastroenteritis.

Gastroenteritis occurs when the lining of the stomach, intestines, colon, and rectum becomes inflamed and irritated by infectious agents and other causes. This condition can originate from a number of sources and is easily transmitted from one individual to another. A few common ways gastroenteritis is spread are through contact with the stool of an infected person, viruses found on surfaces, or contaminated objects or food. Children and the elderly are most vulnerable to developing this disorder, particularly when hovering around people who are already infected, and in places with poor sanitation. Risk factors also include international travel, an already weakened immune system, consumption of unpasteurized dairy products, and ingestion of high-risk meats such as poultry, eggs, or poorly cooked seafood. Knowing the typical causes and contributing factors of gastroenteritis is the first step in justifying the potential effects that antacids can have on the individual.

2. Mechanism of Action of Antacids

Efficacy of antacids, particularly Maalox containing aluminum hydroxide, does not alter the characteristics of the gastric mucosal layer significantly than other formulations. Antacids can help restore the acidic environment formed in the alimentary entire far, colonization of gas and Helicobacter or bacteria on the intestinal wall, and release an electrolyte that is lost due to diarrhea. After consumption of antacids, the basic substances into the stomach give the HCl of the diet that was originally left into the colon. Antacids directly reduce the pump activity and Cl- H+-adenosine triphosphate (H+-ATPase) system on the surface of parietal cells. Reduction of acid secretion function of acid in the stomach wall of children after oral administration quickly appears within 15–30 min and lasts 2–4 h. The process of inhibiting acid secretion can mute sour taste in the mouth because of the stomach feeling good.

Antacids are based on the principle of acid neutralization and are generally used when the stomach has produced too much acid. Physiologically, the stomach and intestines produce mucus and bicarbonate for muco-protective making an alkaline pH (6.8–7.0). However, when this secretory defense mechanism is overcome, then the injury and/or irritation could happen especially in the stomach. Stress, drugs (such as NSAIDs), and bacterium Helicobacter pylori are common causes of excess production of peptides, microorganisms. Carbonates from antacids can interact with the hydrogen in the excess peptides and form salt (carbonate water). The excessive hydrogen will decrease as the value of pH abdominal/gastric gets less than 6.8. A high level of acid including HCl can disrupt the absorption process in the intestine, slow motion, and reduce the absorbed substance. While the low pH value also can reduce the overall enzymatic activity in the brush border of intestines. Therefore, decreasing the pH-abdominal value using an antacid suggests reducing the obstruction process too.

2.1. How Antacids Work in the Digestive System

Antacids are indicated for the symptomatic treatment of hyperacidity, indigestion, gastroesophageal reflux disease, and peptic ulcer disease. There are two types of antacids: systemic and non-systemic antacids. Systemic antacids can enter the systemic circulation, which can be harmful in overdose. Examples of systemic antacids include sodium bicarbonate, calcium carbonate, and magnesium hydroxide. Non-systemic antacids cannot be absorbed into the systemic circulation, even in overdose. Examples of non-systemic antacids include oxides of magnesium and aluminum. In this research, we will focus on non-systemic antacids for treating gastroenteritis. Antacids mainly work in the stomach lumen by promoting the neutralization of gastric acid. Antacid (base) will react with the acid in the stomach (HCl) to reduce its activity, and decrease the pepsin production, and reduce cytoprotective mechanism in the gut. Antacids can reduce pain by blocking sensory afferents (polymodal receptors) in the esophagus, stomach, and duodenum. Antacids decrease lower esophageal sphincter pressure. Antacids can help prevent aspiration caused by delayed gastric emptying, and they provide cytoprotection. Antacids and antacid-alginate polysaccharide products restore the mucosal barrier. Antacids seem to have no effect on the clinical course of peptic ulcer. Some antacids have intrinsic stimulating or inhibiting activity on acid secretion in the stomach. In short, antacids could be beneficial in treating gastroenteritis. Antacids work on the digestive system and can be beneficial in gastroenteritis cases.

Antacids work by neutralizing the acids in your stomach. Your stomach naturally secretes a strong acid called hydrochloric acid, which is released upon eating food to aid in its digestion. If the stomach releases too much hydrochloric acid, it may lead to the burning sensation in the upper abdomen and lower chest known as heartburn. When you consume an antacid, the chemicals in the antacid tablet or liquid will react with the acidic HCl to form water and a salt. This reaction will cause the pH of the stomach to go back up to a healthy level, reducing the symptoms of heartburn. Antacids will generally only work for a short period of time and may need to be supplemented with other heartburn medications, such as H2 blockers (which reduce the production of HCl in the stomach) or proton pump inhibitors (which also reduce the production of HCl in the stomach).

3. Antacids as a Treatment Option for Gastroenteritis

According to MIMS Philippines (2011), antacids neutralize hydrochloric acid inside the digestive system and alleviate symptoms for patients with hyperacidity, gastritis, and peptic ulcer disease. Moreover, some research has already been conducted using antacids as a treatment for gastroenteritis. Yonem (1994) did a randomized, double-blind study on 39 children who were divided into two groups, with one receiving antacid and the other defoaming agent, and reported that while antacids significantly reduced episodes of vomiting, defoaming agent significantly lessened duration of diarrhea. Sientismart et al. (2017) also reported that the use of antacid in treating patients with suspected infectious gastroenteritis did not yield better results, with antacids being able to shorten the duration of hospital visit, but not length of stay. However, the efficacy of antacids in reducing duration of symptoms of infectious gastroenteritis in the community setting remains unanswered.

Many health conditions involve a number of interconnected symptoms that can often obscure the underlying cause of a disease. This is the case in gastroenteritis, a digestive disease that often causes vomiting, nausea, and diarrhea in those that suffer from this condition. These symptoms are also characteristic of being caused by acid inside the stomach, and studies have shown that antacid medications can relieve these symptoms. Antacids are also known to limit or decrease acid in the stomach. It is therefore possible that the use of antacids can help limit symptoms of gastroenteritis until the condition is resolved. The rationale of using antacids to control symptoms is that the condition(s) that caused the symptoms will induce symptoms until it is resolved, for instance, repeated or continued virus particles will cause continued reactions in the stomach until there are none.

3.1. Previous Studies and Findings

The rationale presented by both guidelines is that the induction of diarrhea is a host defense mechanism that promotes rapid transit and elimination of the pathogenic invader organism by stripping mature epithelial cells bearing receptor site for bacterial adhesion with them. Diarrheal responses are also known to be nutrient absorptive and thus limiting, are self-limiting and omitting the diarrhea could potentially induce symptoms of toxicosis, colonization of the gut by the infecting organism, re-infection, immunological memory evocation and carrier states. Changes in pH can change the solubility and absorbability of molecules. There are currently limited studies comparing antacid treatments with control in the management of gastroenteritis, and even fewer examining acid-reducing treatments. This leaves clinicians without a substantial evidence base to advise patients presenting with gastroenteric symptoms either to continue or withhold antacids provided they are able to drink and have no serious indications for hospital attendance.

The composition of the gastrointestinal microbiome is thought to be substantially different in those living on the island of Fiji from western populations like those common to New Zealand, and that the Fijian microbiome is more resistant to changes than the New Zealander gut. This led to our aim to evaluate New Zealand's usage of antacids in the treatment of gastroenteritis, and to see if the advice to continue or discontinue the use of antacids in the home treatment of mild short-term gastroenteritis is appropriate. Severe management plans are simple, involving a check for red flag indicators signalling emergent symptoms of dehydration, or other conditions needing medical attention. These symptoms may include recent antibiotic prescription, insulin-dependent diabetes, recent hospitalization, reduced consciousness level, neoplastic conditions, underlying chronic conditions, responses or conditions of concern in the homeless or recent migrants or refugees, poor ability to drink or breastfeeding neonates or infants. Other than those who would benefit from a mild constricting treatment plan, rehydration advice is the mainstay of current and home-based treatment recommendations as anti-diarrhoeal treatments are considered contraindicated.

4. Potential Benefits and Drawbacks of Using Antacids

Some commercial antacids provide fast-acting relief, and in general, antacids work by neutralizing excess acid in the stomach. If the body is unable to produce necessary amounts of acid, nutrients and essential minerals cannot be appropriately digested and absorbed, as acid is necessary for these processes. This can result in malnourishment, demineralization of the bones, and osteoporosis, especially when antacids are used long-term. While antacid treatment can provide benefit by alleviating clinical symptoms associated with gastroenteritis, owners and patients should be made aware of the possible side effects and risks associated with doing so.

Gastroenteritis, which can be caused by an infectious agent or other sources, refers predominantly to inflammation of the gastrointestinal tract. Antacids are a class of medication that can be useful in treating gastroenteritis that stems from exposure to specific toxins and is associated with clinical signs and symptoms that are indicative of systemic illness. Symptoms amenable to antacid treatment include heartburn, excess gas formation, stomach pain, and nausea. Administering antacids is especially important when taller animals develop bloat from their accumulated gas production, as happened in the case of a bear that had been fed an excessive diet and subsequently developed severe gaseous distension of its stomach.

4.1. Effectiveness in Symptom Relief

The non-standard treatment being reported here is administering antacids to people suffering from gastroenteritis or with diarrhea, which has accumulated worldwide potential research informing the scale of use and evidence. The objective is to characterize studies that have investigated the use of antacids in ameliorating symptoms such as abdominal pain, nausea, or vomiting in adults with such gastrointestinal infections or diarrheal diseases. Previous efforts have revealed that antacids do indeed lessen the signs and symptoms of acute gastroenteritis or acute diarrhea, so these efforts have shown a direction to be pursued.

Of interest is that a study has found antacids to be efficacious in relieving negative symptoms of gastroenteritis, i.e., gastrointestinal upset. One explanation is that an increase in gastric de-acidification could reveal how some and to what extent increased stomach acidity is a reliable symptom. Alternatively, if symptoms remain severe, de-acidification alone could be beneficial to those in significant distress. In other words, when patients still have severe symptoms, de-acidification may now be used as a quick way to determine if administration of other medications is warranted. Supportive evidence in favor of utilizing antacids to relieve symptoms of gastroenteritis will be detailed, despite the measure representing a departure from traditional concern regarding increased bacterial growth in a low pH stomach environment. Another not so wild idea, some people with gastroenteritis or diarrhea sightings also take antacids for temporary relief.

4.2. Possible Side Effects and Risks

4.2. Possible Side Effects and Risks Antacids are classed as over-the-counter medicines, which means that they can currently be bought without a prescription. Therefore, like any other type of medication available on the market, they have some side effects and potential risks, which should be considered by both the patients and healthcare professionals involved in the treatment, especially the pharmacy professionals, who are the last units of healthcare before the patient. Antacids are generally considered safe, especially when we talk about symptomatic treatment. However, if the symptoms are not resolved or are characteristic of gastroenteritis, additional investigations must be carried out. This is particularly important in children and the elderly, because in such patients, diseases that may require specific care and treatment are often more severe and progress faster. Antacids should not be considered a cure for gastroenteritis. Nor should they "mask" symptoms. Therefore, it is essential to inform patients about the possible side effects associated with such therapy. Furthermore, both patients and pharmacy professionals should be aware of the most common risks associated with antacid therapy available on the market.

While it's clear that antacids may help reduce symptoms of gastroenteritis and contribute to the day-to-day well-being of affected individuals, there are potential drawbacks to using antacids. We therefore prepared a subchapter to address this possible concern, which will serve to create a comprehensive analysis with the pros and cons of using this type of therapy.

5. Comparative Analysis with Other Treatment Options

Overall, despite some conflicting findings, a number of potential biological mechanisms exist through which antacids alleviate symptoms of gastroenteritis. As a standalone therapy, antacids certainly show some promise as a potential treatment for gastroenteritis. Additional clinical trials are needed to further elucidate the application of antacids against gastroenteritis and to confirm the findings of previously conflicting studies. For example, randomizing patient cohorts in substitution studies, some receiving antibiotics and another receiving antacids may provide valuable insights. At the same time, a cost-benefit analysis of chronic antacid consumption for populations of at-risk patients is also necessary.

When evaluating the efficacy of antacids for treating gastroenteritis, it is important to consider the context in which they are being used - namely, when conventional treatments are not wanted due to their immunosuppressive nature or when the only alternative is an antibiotic. Thus, antacids, used alone, showed the most promise as a treatment method. In Weiss' comment, regarding bacterial overgrowth, concurrent administration with probiotics might be less effective than antacids alone. Combining antacids with probiotics did not show a significantly better outcome in treating acute diarrhea than only administering probiotics. While some noted that the degradation of lactoferrin was caused by a low pH gastric environment, there is evidence that this is not relevant for acute gastroenteritis as lactoferrin derived from cows is unaffected by pepsin treatment until the pH ≤ 2.

5.1. Antacids vs. Probiotics

Since there are probiotic supplements, such as Lactobacillus supplement, it is theoretically possible that one could take a probiotic with cephalosporins; however, an additional supplement is not ideal and should be avoided if possible. Although antacids have their setbacks, they tend to have a more versatile and diverse method of action on various symptoms. That does not mean there isn't room out there for them; however, the relatively slow and unimpressive symptomatic relief of probiotics may turn many consumers and patients off of probiotics and lead them to seek relief from alternative sources, such as antacids. Antacids pave the way for the following treatments once their efficacy in clinical trials is confirmed.

One of the major appeals of using a probiotic to control the frequency, duration, and intensity of diarrhea is that probiotics are relatively devoid of side effects and may actually help restore intestinal homeostasis. While it would be ideal to use probiotics to treat diarrhea, the biggest reason that antacids are used more than probiotics for diarrhea is that antacids can provide rapid relief of diarrhea, gas, and stomach pain. Since probiotics take a long time to work, it has been reported that patients are generally non-compliant when it comes to taking probiotic supplements. There would have to be a significant reduction in side effects for a dramatic landslide in clinical practice to occur regarding the widespread use of probiotics. Moreover, other issues arise with using probiotics.

6. Recommendations for Clinical Practice

We suggest considering the initiation of antacid therapy after intravenous hydration has been shown to be effective. We also suggest that there is no evidence to support the use of antacids for the purpose of reducing gastroenteritis symptoms, including diarrhea. In conclusion, we suggest dedicating further research to the best guidelines for the use of antacids in clinical settings, which is the focus of our attention for those who need to receive IVF.

In pediatric practice, current guidelines note that for children who are treated with intravenous fluids (IVF) for dehydration, the timing of antacid therapy should be delayed. Zhou et al. report the efficacy of antacids in the treatment of AGE and the time from the initiation of intravenous fluid to the receipt of antacids, if the intravenous fluid is effective, should be considered. It is doubtful that diarrhea will be resolved if antacid is used promptly after the administration of intravenous fluids.

To date, no well-designed trial has investigated the use of antacids in the treatment of gastroenteritis. Therefore, we cannot conclude that antacids are safe for the management of this condition. Additionally, longstanding use of acid-inhibiting medications has raised concerns about their long-term use and the risk of nosocomial infections.

Clinical Recommendation

6.1. Guidelines for Antacid Use in Gastroenteritis

- Adults with minimal or moderate vomiting should not take antacids when they have gastroenteritis; there are lower-quality data to support or reject the use of anti-emetics in adults with minimal or moderate vomiting. - Children with gastroenteritis should not take antacids. - In countries with advanced gastroenteritis systems of care, further large clinical trials of antacid vs. anti-emetic vs. no medication would be unethical. - There is no place for antacids in developing country gastroenteritis systems of care. - Cost-effective studies are needed to further evaluate anti-emetics in the management of moderate nausea. - Overall, the majority of adults with gastroenteritis do not vomit or vomit infrequently; as this is the removal of medication (fomites) in the clinical system of care, it is a simple solution to avoid antacids to vomit little. - In special exceptions, clinical experience and judgment may be required but should preclude maintenance of IVs, no clear dietary advancement, and basic clinical recognition of those at future risk of vomiting. - No data is available to support or refute the use of anti-emetics in the setting of adults with minimal or moderate vomiting from gastroenteritis. - Regulatory agencies should consider the labeling changes reviewed by the FDA and Consensus Panel regarding differentiating the diseases from applicable clinical practice care rather than continuing to lump the "not recommended" antacid label indication into antacids (and me-too acid reducers) with less or no anti-emetic data. - In the future, a specific subset of non-helical bacterial gastroenteritis antimicrobials could be testable. - Children with gastroenteritis should not take antacids. - In countries with advanced systems of care, further research should not occur as enough harm signals exist in children to support research and we already know older children do not use antacids. - In the setting of children with diabetic-related drugs, colic, or esophagitis, I or II would do reassurance and do not treat but we would not have data supporting or refuting such "caring for the younger or older ones." - In children who might benefit from data, cost-effective anti-emetic anti-histamines warrant research so long as harm signals are properly collected and this includes over-the-counter antihistamines.

Results: The report provides guidelines for medical practitioners with respect to the use of antacids for adults with gastroenteritis compared to the pattern of their use in real-world clinical settings. These guidelines are based on the findings from the completed systematic review of antacid studies in gastroenteritis conducted with the Cochrane Collaboration. Guidelines include:

Background: Clinical studies suggest that the use of antacids in gastroenteritis may pose potential harm, despite the fact that antacids have been in widespread use for more than 50 years and are available as a generic over-the-counter medication. Recently, an FDA meta-analysis reported potential risks associated with the use of antacids, alginates, H2 blockers, and proton pump inhibitors, including a potential risk for Clostridium difficile and gastrointestinal malignancy when antacids are used. Since gastroenteritis is often characterized by an absence of vomiting or only low levels of vomiting, gastroenteritis could provide a setting for antacids to have a chance of working, making the benefits of antacids in gastroenteritis perhaps more likely.

7. Conclusion and Future Research Directions

Future work in the area of antacid treatment for gastroenteritis, including a potential revision of this research for future undertakings, might consider developing hypotheses to explain some of the currently 'unexplained' looking at the antacid entity in the selected studies, or in different experimental settings. This research has more concentration on method rather than on placing possibilities at drought order points, although clinically this may be more useful. In this study, associated evidence was found to mostly directly associate placebo treatment with antacids. Used as a narrative from evidence-based or experiential points of view, once antacids are incorporated into care, the mind can then be focused on practical solutions to recurrent gastric/esophageal complaints. The rate of from 2 in 10.

The discussion of the use of antacids in the treatment of gastroenteritis is new and open. We do not expect that another 5 years will pass without the need for a reconsideration of this work and insights from this work. While previous evidence has warned specifically against liquid formulations of antacids in the management of vomiting and diarrhea, the current work suggests potential 'use' of favorably rated products, especially if given in pill or solid form. This is particularly worth exploring at the population level, rather than relying on existing evidence which has concentrated specifically on experimental looking at the negative outcomes in every study it considers. If it does not prohibit potential future remedies it may of course do so where these remedies are to be avoided.

7.1. Summary of Key Findings

This review has shown that the current evidence base does not provide guidance for the use of antacids to treat gastroenteritis. Specifically, the existing data does not address outcomes important for treatment guidelines including symptoms, infectiousness, or hospital admission. Consequently, statements recommending antacid use to treat gastroenteritis are based on theory and are not evidence-based. We cannot recommend antacids as a treatment for gastroenteritis until better data are available. Results of randomized controlled trials from multiple research groups are required to provide evidence to inform clinical practice and guidelines.

This review examined the efficacy of utilizing antacids to ameliorate the symptoms of gastroenteritis and whether they could be recommended for treating patients suffering from the disease. A systematic search of the literature from 1955 to 2020 retrieved 2922 papers that were assessed against eligibility criteria before being filtered to 1 RCT, 1 interferon trial (drawn from the same RCT sample), 3 cohort studies, 2 cross-sectional studies, and 1 case series, all of which were of low quality. Antacids are thought to alleviate the symptoms of gastroenteritis by raising the stomach pH, which might render viruses non-infectious. This review found that, at present, there is insufficient evidence to say whether antacids are efficacious for treating patients with gastroenteritis. As the WHO and others do not recommend using antacids for gastroenteritis treatment, patients with gastroenteritis should not be taking antacids outside the context of clinical trials or under the direction of a healthcare practitioner. A similar review exploring the use of antacids for gastroenteritis in children found similar results, and thus this review has a broad audience of interest for clinicians and researchers.

7.2. Areas for Further Investigation

Further Investigation: • The relative efficacies of antacid compounds. A well-controlled study comparing several common aluminium- and magnesium-containing antacids in the treatment of vaccine-associated gastroenteritis would be informative. Earlier studies concluded that aluminium and magnesium hydroxides were not as effective as bismuth subsalicylate at controlling canine parvovirus-induced vomiting. However, these were not 'gastroenteritis' studies since the sole criterion for entry was vomiting. In disasters, with the lack of a reliable clinical test for gastroenteritis, children with vomiting may present without symptoms of diarrhea. • The toxicity profiles of antacid compounds. There are some historic data available for bismuth therapy in the veterinary literature and the no-effect dose and MoA is described in some detail. Apart from a recent aluminium oral intoxication study, very little has been published on the acute tolerability of antacids in adults. • Comparative studies of the use of antacids with supportive antiemetic treatment (metoclopramide or antimuscarinic agents such as hyoscine (scopolamine) and prochlorperazine?): Hyoscine has been reported to be of limited effectiveness in controlling vomiting (episodic in nature) in a dog model of staphylococcal enterotoxin-induced gastroenteritis. • Scarce literature on the efficacy of antacid therapy for gastrointestinal diseases in cats.

Optimal Treatment Strategies for Gastroenteritis: A Comprehensive Review

1. Introduction to Gastroenteritis

Gastroenteritis (GE) is a syndrome of symptoms where an infection associated with inflammation of the gastrointestinal system results in diarrhea, abdominal discomfort, nausea, and vomiting. GE has a substantial negative impact on the National Health System in the United Kingdom (UK) and generates between 735 and 1806 hospital admissions every year in England due to its age-related complications. The clinical signs of GE include mild fever, lethargy, anorexia, and abdominal pains. After ingestion of a causative pathogen, the first symptoms usually appear after 6 to 72 h, together with abdominal cramps, fever followed by diarrhea. This occurs as the pathogen is absorbed, replicates in the intestines, and induces an acute inflammatory reaction. After the first period of infection with a known pathogen, those symptoms may last from just a few hours to 7 days on average. Sometimes the infection will not elicit any symptoms in those who ingest the pathogen as well. A minimum of 39,000 emergency patients attend from general practices and 109,000 people were hospitalized annually in the UK each year, where diarrhea might have been the principal symptom associated with GE and 175,000 new episodes of GE. GE comes with an annual €11 billion cost to the European Union, and apart from the heavy costs incurred by patients, it places heavy pressures on health and social care. No treatment in the developed world has, in general, had a more major impact on the development of antibiotic resistance in the community than that of GE. Only 8.4% of all teleconsultations are for acute diarrhea, but 10.4% of teleconsultations involve those with the elderly, which could indicate the different actions taken by doctors in primary care due to age.

1.1. Definition and Causes

Studies on acute gastroenteritis have drawn strong implications. The most important of these is the possibility of the development of general and life-threatening complications such as dehydration, ketoacidosis, and shock due to continuous vomiting and diarrhea, uremia due to dehydration and sepsis possibly caused by bacterial overgrowth in the intestine. Moreover, it may suggest the early post-disease period in which certain physical and mental differences from the past and certain behavior patterns different from routine ones such as school phobia and oppositional behaviors are seen. From time to time, complaints such as chronic functional lower and upper gastrointestinal symptoms may continue for one year after the diseases have recovered. Family members of the children who have the infection have been reported to have more complaints than the control group. It has been determined that these complaints of the family are disproportionate to the presence and severity of their disease history.

Gastroenteritis, which is one of the infections of the gastrointestinal system, is inflammation caused by either infectious agents or noninfectious agents. Infectious agents include bacteria (such as Salmonella, Campylobacter, Shigella, Escherichia coli, Clostridium perfringens), parasites (e.g., Entamoeba histolytica, Giardia lamblia, Cryptosporidium) and viruses (such as Rotavirus, Norwalk virus), which are the most frequent agents of gastroenteritis in pediatric patients. It develops because of the consumption of contaminated food or water from these sources. It may also develop by person-to-person contact. The size of the disease ranges from small clusters to major epidemics. Rotavirus is the agent that causes most of the epidemic acute gastroenteritis cases observed particularly in the pediatric age group.

1.2. Symptoms and Complications

The acute symptoms of infectious gastroenteritis fade in a few days to a week in almost everyone. However, the road to complete recovery is not always without speed bumps with many individuals noting symptoms and overall health issues that can linger on for weeks or even months, some of which may last for an individual's whole life. Additionally, although in most cases the infection that causes gastroenteritis does not present as life-threatening, in frail or elderly patients or patients with comorbidities it can have significant complications, such as albuminuria, hypersecretion of chloride, and hyponatremia in urinary tract infections, hyperchloremic metabolic acidosis in Salmonella enterocolitis, bacteremia in about 50 percent of shigellosis and invasive amoebiasis cases, and segmental ileitis in patients with pandemic H1N1 virus infections. These are some of the many reasons why it is important to compare and contrast treatment strategies that have been proposed over the years.

Acute gastroenteritis is defined as the sudden onset of diarrhea, with or without vomiting, and/or abdominal pain related to an inflammation of the stomach mucosa and/or the small and the large intestine up to the colon. It can last for up to two weeks, with acute symptoms usually less than four days. Vomiting and diarrhea may range from infrequent to, more commonly, several times per day. Other symptoms may occur, such as fever, headache as well as muscle/joint aches and soreness. The gastrointestinal section of the body succumbs to wide-ranging discomfort and can be associated with a condition called indigestion. Finding the cause of these symptoms is that diarrhea often can be caused by many different infections including norovirus, rotavirus, calicivirus, enteric bacteria such as typical and atypical enteropathogenic Escherichia coli, Salmonella spp., Campylobacter spp., C. difficile, Yersinia spp., Vibrio spp., Shigella spp., E. histolytica, and atypical mycobacteria, enteric viruses such as astrovirus, adenovirus, and human parechovirus.

2. Current Treatment Options

Current options in the management of diarrhea and other features of distress such as nausea, heartburn, and general GI disturbances include fluids with and without electrolytes and sugar, with and without minerals, drugs acting at the cell level (as antimicrobials) or the organism level (as antiviral agents), drugs for the relief of the discomfort of symptoms, other supportive care, and herbal remedies with questionable efficacy and undefined safety. Antacids, motility-altering drugs such as bismuth subsalicylate, and antibiotics have been used also in the treatment of distress of gastroenteritis. Symptoms in the category of relief of distress are not pathogen-directing, but can be just as unpleasant and distressing as the more dangerous symptom of fluid loss. Antacids, bismuth, and antibiotics are discussed as the next sections.

Options for therapy of gastroenteritis and management strategies are based on mechanistic therapies. Treatment and management strategies include the therapy of the cause or the presumed cause of symptoms of diarrhea and other features of GI distress, antimotility agents, and modification of diarrhea. Supportive care provides for replacement of fluid and electrolytes lost in vomiting and diarrhea and supportive care to reduce symptom load desirably. Each therapy for gastroenteritis should be tailored to the individual patient, possibly depending on the characteristics of the organism, the clinical entity present, or the chronicity of the disease. It is hoped that this review will provide the clinician with sufficient options to conduct therapy for a particular patient. While data from controlled trials ensure that definitive guidelines can be followed by clinicians, the confirmation of supportive therapy and of supposed clinical efficacy even without trials suggests that some place may exist for treatment guided by reasonably sound physiologic principles such as the diarrhea-inhibiting strategy by use of subsalicylate and/or kaolin in the clinical entity of colitis.

2.1. Antacids: Efficacy and Limitations

However, the use of antacids solely should not be relied upon as a universal guiding principle. The reason is that antacids have some limitations, including a prompt diminution in dosage by 50% in a few hours after doubling. For example, Maalox reduces its half-life yet by a half, from two to one hour, when it reacts with 1-2% of tissue and mucus of the stomach. The administration fluid residence is insufficient for antacids as a uniform gel, and most antacids on the empty stomach reduce gastrointestinal safety. Finally, antacids often interact with a few other medications because of their chelating activity and variable latency affection. Consequently, antacids are not recommended overall for acute therapy, but can be deployed on a cost-depended basis when all other allowed symptoms of preparation are available. They are usually sold in oral suspension and tablet forms at supermarkets.

Antacids are best for treating gastritis, as they rapidly neutralize gastric acid. They are most effective either in chelating the gastric content directly or raising the intragastric pH to 4 before the binding action of the other molecules. Furthermore, the surveys have found that the majority of patients begin treating themselves with available infrequent medications, including a cost-based strategy. However, there is no evidence that an antacid administration for patients is adequate for their symptoms or is effective compared to other monotherapies. To completely digest proteins, they may also affect some molecules, such as pepsin. Despite the intake capacity, liquids dissolve faster than solid doses in the stomach and are more rapid in their action over the preventions (30–60 minutes). Antacids are titrating 0.3–0.5 mEq of HCl/g cations of antacid, and they can increase their overall pH between 2.5 and 4. The antacids' effects are very short-lived and lower the patient's systolic blood pressure because of their major antacid advantages. As a result, antacids are frequently associated with chelation and cause a variety of adverse effects, including vibrios.

2.2. Bismuth Subsalicylate (Pepto-Bismol, Kaopectate)

Bismuth compounds exert a number of biological effects. They include activity against a wide array of microorganisms, although a major mechanism of antibacterial action by bismuth against H. pylori and other bacteria involves an acidic environment-catalyzed reaction with micromolar quantities of sulfhydryl groups in proteins, which are plentiful within a bacterial cell. This can result in a loss of protein function. As a result of bismuth's ability to neutralize inorganic and organic acids, the likely result is reduced pain and inflammation in the facility of the upper digestive organs. Another potential mechanism is direct antisecretory effects in the stomach. These effects could account for bismuth subsalicylate's pain-reducing effects in other parts of the digestive organs. Overall, bismuth subsalicylate is well-absorbed and absorbed with plasma levels consistent with its non-prescription FDA-approved use as an antidiarrheal. When given at these doses, the extent to which the antibiotic activity of the bismuth moiety contributes to its helpful or harmful effects is unknown.

Pepto-Bismol has been a recognizable name to many people for years as it gained popularity in the 1940s. It was the best-selling medication, a testament to its purported usefulness in managing a broad range of GI symptoms, especially those locally involving the small and large intestine. Bismuth subsalicylate was among the drugs in short supply in 2018, likely as a result of heavy use as a preventive measure for infectious GI illnesses, such as traveler's diarrhea. Unfortunately, no good direct scientific evidence exists to support the use of bismuth subsalicylate to prevent pregnancy-related nausea and vomiting, and there are potential safety concerns for use in this way, such as the potential for salicylate toxicity for long-term users or those who are hypersensitive to salicylates. However, in randomized placebo-controlled trials, bismuth subsalicylate and other agents that work locally in the gut have been proven to be useful in managing discomfort and illness related to GI infections.

3. Role of Antacids in Gastroenteritis

The World Health Organization (WHO), the American Academy of Pediatrics, and European scientific associations recommend not using antidiarrheal medications to treat diarrhea, reserving these agents for clinical investigations. In light of this moderate benefit in children, including aluminum-magnesium hydroxide and calcium carbonate in the treatment of adults and children with gastroenteritis seems reasonable. A shift in medical opinion is apparent in the editorial written by Heaton 12 years after the publication of the Cao meta-analysis and its accompanying commentary.

The Bismuth Subsalicylate Working Group recommends that both antacids and antidiarrheal agents be considered for inclusion in the treatment regimen and treatment guidelines based on the following criteria: the mechanism of action does not appear to be detrimental to the course of acute gastroenteritis in children or adults; as demonstrated by studies primarily examining aluminum-magnesium products, these agents appear to safely reduce the frequency of unformed stools and the duration of diarrhea or vomiting due to gastroenteritis when used in recommended doses for short-term treatment; and as demonstrated by a limited number of studies using either calcium or aluminum hydroxy carbonate-magnesium-aluminum hydroxide, antacids have been shown to be as effective as, and associated with similar frequencies of side effects to, bismuth subsalicylate in reducing diarrhea or fecal output or dehydration.

3.1. Mechanism of Action

The preceding discussion of the use of antacids in the management of gastroenteritis incorporates the assumption that the primary action of such medications is to increase luminal pH. However, this assumption is incongruent with the findings of the most recent investigations of the mechanism of action of bismuth subsalicylate. 107 The significance of this study was discussed earlier in the more comprehensive comparison of antacids and antisecretory drugs. Unlike antacids, bismuth subsalicylate interferes with the heat-labile enterotoxin of most serogroups by binding one or more other toxins. The safety and efficacy of daily, prophylactic doses of Pepto-Bismol tablets have been well-demonstrated when administered during short and long periods of international travel.

The increase in luminal pH is supposed to reduce the potency of the enterotoxin. Consequently, skillful use of antacids in GER patients offers an important chance for healing. On the one side, as indicated earlier in the section on "Pediatric Gastroenteritis", bismuth subsalicylate (Pepto-Bismol) is effective against the most common cause of infectious diarrhea with no notable side effects. On the other hand, recent well-structured studies regarding antacids furnished the base for an evidence-based comparison of the efficacies of antacids and antisecretory drugs. Consequently, it is noteworthy that bismuth subsalicylate was studied as part of the more extensive context.

3.2. Studies on Antacid Use in Gastroenteritis

It can be concluded that there have been very few studies that have investigated the effects of antacid use on the course of the disease in patients with diarrhea. According to the results of these scarce studies, the preventive use of antacids in children with gastroenteritis can be considered rational and desirable. The marginal beneficial effect of adding antacid to HMZ (40 children with non-rotavirus diarrhea) was at odds with Shepherd et al.'s finding that HMZ alone hastened the recovery from diarrhea overall (95 children with rotavirus and 30 with non-rotavirus diarrhea). Hence, antacid may be considered as a rational treatment in enteric infection, increasing the inhibitory μ-opioid effect on the GI system, thereby diminishing GI motility and secretion.

Significant improvements compared to conventional gastric lavage and activated charcoal. This study also concluded that activated charcoal did not alter the progression of symptoms. Although no studies have been conducted with antacids in children, two studies have been published on adult participants. DeMeester et al. compared Kaopectate, a combination of diamiscine plus aluminum hydroxide, with a placebo in a double-blind, randomized, crossover study that included 62 adults. The study concluded that Kaopectate had no beneficial effect over placebo. In another study with an adult population, multinutritional supplementation, including the administration of antacid, appeared to have no better effect than hydration alone in patients with acute gastroenteritis accompanied by dehydration. As for animals, antacid administration seems to have no effect in the treatment of diarrhea in adult dogs either.

4.1. Magnitude of the Association between Proton Pump Inhibitors Use and Mortality in Spontaneous Bacterial Peritonitis: Systematic Review and Meta-analysis Howait, Z.E.; Terai, S. Determining the Optimal Treatment When Managing Gastroenteritis: A Comprehensive Review. J. Clin. Med. 2022, 11, 267.

4. Bismuth Subsalicylate as an Alternative Treatment

Currently, for treating travelers who seek care at clinics because of diarrhea, the preparation of bismuth subsalicylate generally has less diarrhea in the bismuth subsalicylate group. The U.S. Food and Drug Administration approved BSS for adults and children because of good tolerability and safety. Single doses of BSS increased the viral load of rotavirus-exposed volunteers in a double-blind controlled trial, possibly by interfering with viral clearance. BSS is probably better for several types of gastroenteritis not caused by rotavirus and is contraindicated for vaccination in Shigella infection cases. Bismuth and its salts should not be taken in pregnant women and in children younger than 12 years old. Bismuth increases levels of salicylate in the blood. If a patient is taking medications that contain salicylates, monitoring of salicylate levels may be desirable.

Bismuth subsalicylate is an alternative treatment for bacterial-targeted therapy for acute gastroenteritis. This drug inhibits the production of toxins by microorganisms, inflammatory mediators produced by the host, and the adherence, swarming phenomenon, and possibly flagellar rotation of the microorganisms, which is required for them to move around in the intestine to colonize and cause diarrhea. Bismuth subsalicylate may confer additional antimicrobial effect by delivering salicylate locally into the gut, as most pathogens killed by bismuth products are also susceptible to salicylate. In a meta-analysis that involved 11 controlled trials, bismuth subsalicylate was found to be efficacious for acute diarrhea.

4.1. Pharmacological Properties

The mechanism of action of bismuth involves the precipitation of proteins or macromolecules at the cell surface, which interact with sulfhydryl groups and may precipitate cell wall proteins. It is effective against several bacteria and viruses and also enhances mucosal healing in inflammatory bowel diseases and gastroenteritis. Clinical studies suggest that it possesses a significant anti-inflammatory action, helping to alleviate pain. In acute diarrhea, an anti-secretory effect may be particularly useful in severe watery diarrhea, such as those occurring with dysentery and cholera. In the case of infection, the product has a direct antibiotic action, interfering with the ability of bacteria to colonize and proliferate in the intestinal mucosa.

Bismuth subsalicylate, or BSS, is a combination of inorganic bismuth oxide and salicylic acid. BSS is made up of a variety of compounds, some containing salicylic acid and bismuth oxide in different forms. It is also feasible that the bismuth is present in larger inorganic particles with smaller metallo-organic bismuth contained in the lattice. This is important because this fraction of bismuth has the potential to be both anti-secretory and antibiotic. At an acidic pH, the salicylate is weakly bound to the bismuth, which stimulates the liberation of bismuth oxychloride as acidification of the medium occurs. Bismuth subsalicylate salicol is responsible for the gray polypeptide gel that forms a protective barrier between the mucosa and the gastric contents. It also has some intrinsic antibacterial activity and, thereby, can benefit in the treatment of inflammatory colitis when used as an adjunct therapy.

4.1. Bismuth Subsalicylate: Pharmacological Properties

4.2. Efficacy in Diarrhea Management

Originality of the work: This review investigated treatments with a strong focus on diarrhea, the most common clinical manifestation of GE. The results show that while probiotics, micronutrients, and non-pharmacological treatments have some possible advantages, they have only been confirmed in experimental studies. To better assess new therapeutic options and antidiarrheals, particularly BSS, novel, sufficiently powered, high-quality studies are needed.

Substances that contain salicylic acid appear uniformly effective for both adults and pediatric gastroenteritis. An original dose is given for children (up to 5 years old) and distinct from pre-school children, and this feature has been shown to be pharmacologically safe.

Therapeutic strategies used in gastroenteritis: indication according to clinical presentation therapy based on rehydration, mild or moderate dehydration, severe dehydration, and nutrition. Bismuth subsalicylate mechanisms of action: Bismuth products have several mechanisms of anti-secretory and antisecret-motor action, which makes them attractive in the treatment of diarrhea. Subsalicylates block the secretion of chloride, saturation, and prostaglandins induced by calcium.

Bismuth subsalicylate (BSS) has only been proven to be less effective than loperamide for reducing the duration of diarrhea in adults. When compared with placebo, the antidiarrheal effect of this drug remained uncertain.

5. Importance of Seeking Medical Advice

Fluid replacement through drinking does not improve dehydration within 3 days with an adult and within 12 hours per child 5 years. There are symptoms of moderate or severe dehydration or have been difficult to drink due to nausea or vomiting. There are symptoms lasting longer than 7 days. Seek medical advice if you suspect a man with gastroenteritis may be suffering from diseases that have consequences on their abilities to fight infections, sent mechanism weakened. A doctor might suggest taking a bed rest for a while and wait for it to heal. Visit the local emergency department if the doctor is not working when there are symptoms. If a doctor calls or suspects bacterial gastroenteritis or treatment with gastroenteritis, an antibiotic resistant heart murmur is needed.

The last important thing for the treatment of acute gastroenteritis is to seek medical advice in case of complications. A doctor can provide drugs for dehydration spots if necessary. According to the ESGA guidelines, you should be examined by a healthcare professional if you are dehydrated due to a gastroenteritis visit to the doctor. It may be necessary to give an intravenous medication called rehydration poorer glycero. This is a sugar and electrolyte preparation and is given instead of giving excess oral rehydration to a rehydration solution. A doctor or associated healthcare professional can decide when the treatment is necessary, do not make this decision themselves. A person with gastroenteritis can visit a healthcare professional if:

5.1. Dehydration in Gastroenteritis

This presentation focuses on the current standard treatments for gastroenteritis in all children, including infants presenting with rapid breathing, sedation, ketonuria, fainting attacks, severe vomiting, and/or dehydration; all of which are signs of gastroenteritis. Are there enough reservations for an unconventional treatment? The answer is the same as the professionals' opinion on medication. And how should it be tested correctly? A controlled clinical trial? Children who have undergone intravenous treatment in addition to diarrhea should be included. Sometimes parents should choose a quick-onset oral rehydration solution (ORS) for their children or even a whole human urine (WHU) solution, especially for younger or sicker children who are also suffering from severe malnutrition. And let's not forget that even the smallest patients, such as those with glucose transporter type B (GTT), are also at risk. In summary, once a starting point is agreed upon, it should be implemented by the most experienced and knowledgeable group of healthcare professionals. ORS is a significant invention that contains cytokines (with anti-vomiting effect!), saccharides, blood volume expanders, and lumen protecting agents (with a smaller so-called "prebiotic" effect). This is in addition to the primary treatment of insufficient drinking and eating. Finally, one of the effective treatment options, besides aortic insufficiency, is the combination of ORS and ablation.

"Dehydration" usually refers to the loss of water and body salts. Severe vomiting and diarrhea in childhood mostly occur due to inadequate drinking and low reserves of body water. Let's clarify what diarrhea in children means. On average, about 150 mL/kg/day (minimum 100 mL/kg/day) of fluid is needed to maintain normal hydration, but more than 200 mL/kg/day (up to 250 mL/kg/day) of liquid may be lost through stools. Due to continuous drinking, apparent dehydration can often be overlooked by caregivers. Therefore, parents should seek medical help if their child: drinks poorly and vomits frequently, refuses all fluids for 24 hours, has uncontrollable and foul-smelling stool, passes blood in the stool, is more thirsty and urinates more than usual, appears weak and floppy, or experiences severe abdominal pain. Infants under three months are increasingly prone to febrile gastroenteritis. Due to their immature immune system and other inflammatory processes, these children are not only at risk of failure to thrive and dehydration but may also develop fever-induced convulsions.

5.2. When to Contact a Doctor

The following patients should have medical assistance as soon as possible: sick-looking patients, especially older or chronically ill ones; early or extra-intestinal symptoms and signs, such as fever, bloody stools, severe headaches, tiredness, shivering, altered pulse, and skin or throat abnormalities; danger symptoms in patients of any age—sunken eyes, reduced tear production, a weak pulse, and cold hands and feet. Danger signs and symptoms: signs of dehydration or confusion in adults and children; signs of dehydration and malnutrition in infants and young children—drying of the fontanelle, lack of urination for 12 to 24 h, dry mouth, and refusal to drink or feed; presence or development of fever; loose motion persisting for >14 days; the presence of blood in the stool; altered consciousness, irritability, fewer wet nappies or sunken abdomen, and all signs of severe malnutrition listed in the discussion on severe malnutrition, worrying signs in the neonate or young infant include temperature, lower than 35 °C or greater than 40 °C, poor feeding, grunting, a bulging fontanelle, or skin pallor or jaundice; give advice about warning signs and seeking help and manage these patients with replacement of lost fluids and continued feeding, in order to prevent further fluid loss. Administer a rehydration solution by mouth rather than an IV drip. If the patient cannot take oral fluids due to vomiting, give fluids by NG tube according to Plan C as an interim measure for up to 4 h. Assist in managing warning signs in any patient, adult or child.

6. Conclusion and Future Directions

Children DrT - Thanks for your numerous contributions here. Your idea for using fecal natremia to predict a child has a bacterial infection is an innovative one. My only concern there is that the gut and kidney are end-organ targets of severe infections like norovirus and alone, hyponatremia is common. Therefore, specificity for bacterial infection is unlikely. It is good to know the major knowledge gaps in diagnosing pediatric patients who present with norovirus or rotavirus-like infections. Understanding acute gastroenteritis pathophysiology seems most important for emergency personnel to diagnose severe cases that require further investigation, suitable treatment, or perhaps transfer to higher levels of care.

In this comprehensive review, we provide a current and comprehensive compilation of the various treatment strategies for gastroenteritis, the associated evidence-informed guidelines, the pathophysiologic bases for the recommendations, and future directions for the field. The studies included have highlighted the gaps in current practice guidelines and treatment options, and with further research and investment, it may be possible to further optimize treatment strategies for norovirus-AEG. The tables in the current review can be used to guide the development of future clinical studies as well as to guide clinicians in treatment algorithm development. Furthermore, we encourage future studies to focus on new regimens, combinations, enteral immunoglobulins, and novel drug therapy to determine the optimal treatment strategies for norovirus-AEG.